365 DAYS GUIDE FOR DIABETES:

A Holistic Guide to Wellness and Control

By

Dr. Olivia Harry

Copyright

No part of this book should be copied, reproduced without the author's permission © 2024

TABLE OF CONTENT

Copyright _____ 2

TABLE OF CONTENT _____ 3

CHAPTER ONE _____ 7

DEFINITION AND OVERVIEW OF DIABETES MELLITUS ___ 7

   HISTORICAL PERSPECTIVE OF THE DISEASE ____ 8

CHAPTER TWO _____ 11

UNDERSTANDING THE ENEMY: THE TYPES OF DIABETES MELLITUS _____ 11

   TYPE 1 DIABETES MELLITUS _____ 12

   TYPE 2 DIABETES MELLITUS _____ 13

CHAPTER THREE _____ 15

UNRAVELING THE MYSTERY: CAUSES AND RISK FACTORS FOR DIABETES MELLITUS _____ 15

   GENETIC FACTORS IN DIABETES MELLITUS ____ 17

   LIFESTYLE AND ENVIRONMENTAL FACTORS IN DIABETES MELLITUS _____ 18

OTHER CONTRIBUTING FACTORS IN DIABETES MELLITUS _____ 20

CHAPTER FOUR _____ 23

RECOGNIZING THE ENEMY: SYMPTOMS AND DIAGNOSIS OF DIABETES MELLITUS _____ 23

THE COMMON SYMPTOMS OF DIABETES MELLITUS _____ 25

THE DIAGNOSTIC TESTS FOR DIABETES MELLITUS _____ 27

CHAPTER FIVE _____ 29

THE COMPLICATIONS OF DIABETES MELLITUS _____ 29

SHORT TERM COMPLICATIONS _____ 29

LONG TERM COMPLICATIONS _____ 31

CHAPTER SIX _____ 33

MANAGEMENT AND TREATMENT FOR DIABETES _____ 33

MEDICATIONS _____ 35

INSULIN THERAPY _____ 36

LIFESTYLE CHANGES _____ 38

CHAPTER SEVEN _____ 41

DIET AND NUTRITION FOR DIABETES MELLITUS _____ 41

IMPORTANCE OF HEALTHY EATING IN DIABETES MELLITUS 42

MEAL PLANNING FOR DIABETICS 44

GLYCEMIC INDEX AND GLYCEMIC LOAD 45

CHAPTER EIGHT 47

THE PHYSICAL ACTIVITIES FOR DIABETICS FOR OPTIMAL RECOVERY 47

EXERCISE RECOMMENDATIONS FOR DIABETICS 48

BENEFIT OF REGULAR PHYSICAL ACTIVITY 50

CHAPTER NINE 53

MONITORING BLOOD SUGAR LEVELS 53

HOME MONITORING 55

IMPORTANCE OF REGULAR CHECKS 56

CHAPTER TEN 59

PSYCHOSOCIAL ASPECTS OF DIABETES 59

EMOTIONAL ASPECTS OF DIABETES 61

COPING STRATEGIES FOR DIABETES 63

CHAPTER ELEVEN 67

PREVENTION AND RISK REDUCTION OF DIABETES 67

CHAPTER TWELVE — 71

LIVING WITH DIABETES: OVERCOMING DAILY CHALLENGES — 71

EVERYDAY CHALLENGES — 73

SUPPORT SYSTEMS FOR THOSE LIVING WITH DIABETES — 76

A MESSAGE OF HOPE DESPITE A JOURNEY WITH DIABETES — 78

CHAPTER ONE

DEFINITION AND OVERVIEW OF DIABETES MELLITUS

Diabetes mellitus, commonly known as diabetes, is a chronic metabolic disorder characterized by elevated blood glucose levels, resulting from insufficient insulin production, ineffective utilization of insulin, or a combination of both. Insulin, produced by the pancreas, plays a crucial role in regulating blood sugar levels by facilitating the uptake of glucose into cells for energy. In diabetes, this intricate balance is disrupted, leading to persistent hyperglycemia.

There are two primary types of diabetes: Type 1 and Type 2. Type 1 diabetes is an autoimmune system condition where the immune system erroneously assaults and obliterates insulin-delivering beta cells in the pancreas.. This form typically manifests early in life and requires lifelong insulin replacement therapy. On the other hand, Type 2 diabetes, more prevalent among adults, involves insulin resistance, where the body's cells fail to respond effectively to insulin. Over time, the pancreas may also lose its ability to produce sufficient insulin.

The global prevalence of diabetes has surged in recent decades, attributable to lifestyle changes, sedentary habits, and increasing obesity rates. Unmanaged diabetes can lead to a spectrum of complications, impacting vital organs such as the heart, kidneys, eyes, and nerves. Early diagnosis, lifestyle modifications, and appropriate medical management are crucial in mitigating the impact of diabetes on individuals' health and well-being.

HISTORICAL PERSPECTIVE OF THE DISEASE

The historical perspective of diabetes mellitus traces back to ancient times, with descriptions of symptoms resembling diabetes found in ancient Egyptian manuscripts dating as far back as 1500 BCE. The term "diabetes" itself originates from the Greek word meaning "siphon," a reference to the excessive urination characteristic of the condition.

Throughout history, observations and understanding of diabetes evolved. In the 17th century, Thomas Willis, an English physician, noted the sweet taste of diabetic urine, a key diagnostic clue. However, it wasn't until the early 20th century that significant breakthroughs occurred. In 1921, Canadian scientists Frederick Banting and Charles Best successfully isolated insulin, a hormone crucial for glucose regulation, from the pancreas. This discovery revolutionized diabetes treatment, transforming it from a fatal to a manageable condition.

The classification of diabetes into Type 1 and Type 2 emerged in the latter half of the 20th century, refining our understanding of the disease. Advances in technology, such as the development of glucose monitoring devices and insulin analogs, have further improved diabetes management.

The historical journey of diabetes reflects a gradual unraveling of its complexities, from ancient descriptions to modern scientific breakthroughs, marking a transformative path that has significantly enhanced the quality of life for those living with diabetes.

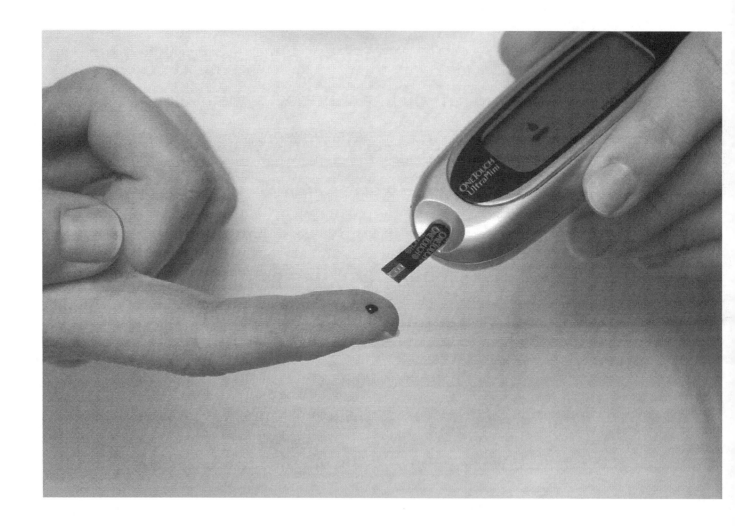

CHAPTER TWO

UNDERSTANDING THE ENEMY: THE TYPES OF DIABETES MELLITUS

Diabetes mellitus encompasses several types, each with distinct characteristics and underlying causes. The two primary types are Type 1 and Type 2:

TYPE 1 DIABETES MELLITUS

Type 1 diabetes is an autoimmune condition characterized by the immune system's misguided attack on the insulin-producing beta cells in the pancreas. This results in a profound deficiency of insulin, the hormone crucial for regulating blood glucose levels. Typically diagnosed in childhood or adolescence, Type 1 diabetes constitutes a smaller percentage of overall diabetes cases. The onset of Type 1 diabetes is often abrupt, marked by symptoms such as excessive thirst, frequent urination, unexplained weight loss, and fatigue. The autoimmune nature of the disease implies a life-long dependence on exogenous insulin, either delivered through injections or an insulin pump, to compensate for the body's inability to produce this vital hormone. Management of Type 1 diabetes involves a delicate balance of insulin administration, blood glucose monitoring, and dietary considerations. Continuous advancements in technology, such as continuous glucose monitoring systems and insulin delivery devices, have significantly improved the quality of life for individuals with Type 1 diabetes. While the exact triggers for the autoimmune response leading to Type 1 diabetes remain under investigation, genetic factors and environmental influences are believed to contribute.

TYPE 2 DIABETES MELLITUS

Type 2 diabetes, the more prevalent form of diabetes mellitus, is characterized by insulin resistance, where the body's cells become less responsive to insulin, and a gradual decline in insulin production by the pancreas. This results in elevated blood glucose levels, a condition known as hyperglycemia. Unlike Type 1 diabetes, Type 2 often develops later in life, although its occurrence in younger individuals is rising, partly due to lifestyle factors. The development of Type 2 diabetes is closely linked to sedentary lifestyles, obesity, and genetic predisposition. Lifestyle factors, including poor dietary habits and physical inactivity, contribute to the development of insulin resistance. Over time, the pancreas struggles to maintain sufficient insulin production, leading to an imbalance in glucose regulation. Management of Type 2 diabetes typically involves lifestyle modifications such as a balanced diet, regular exercise, and weight management. Medications may also be prescribed, ranging from oral drugs that enhance insulin sensitivity to medications that stimulate insulin release. In more advanced cases, insulin therapy might be necessary.

Prevention strategies focus on lifestyle changes, highlighting the importance of healthy eating habits, regular physical activity, and weight control. Type 2 diabetes is a significant global health concern, and its increasing prevalence emphasizes the importance of public health initiatives and individual awareness to curb its impact.

CHAPTER THREE

UNRAVELING THE MYSTERY: CAUSES AND RISK FACTORS FOR DIABETES MELLITUS

The causes and risk factors of diabetes mellitus are multifaceted, involving a complex interplay of genetic, environmental, and lifestyle elements. Here's an overview:

1. Genetic Factors: A family history of diabetes increases the risk, suggesting a genetic predisposition. Certain gene variants may contribute to both Type 1 and Type 2 diabetes.

2. Autoimmune Response (Type 1):

In Type 1 diabetes, an autoimmune reaction triggers the immune system to attack and destroy insulin-producing beta cells in the pancreas. The exact triggers remain under investigation.

3. Insulin Resistance (Type 2):

The primary cause of Type 2 diabetes is insulin resistance, where cells become less responsive to insulin. This resistance is often associated with obesity, sedentary lifestyles, and poor dietary choices.

4. Obesity and Lifestyle:

Excess body weight, especially abdominal obesity, increases the risk of Type 2 diabetes. Unhealthy diets rich in refined sugars and saturated fats contribute to weight gain and insulin resistance.

5. Age and Ethnicity:

Age is a non-modifiable risk factor, with the risk of Type 2 diabetes increasing with age. Certain ethnic groups, including African Americans, Hispanic/Latino Americans, and Native Americans, are more susceptible.

6. Gestational Diabetes:

Women who experience gestational diabetes during pregnancy have an elevated risk of developing Type 2 diabetes later in life.

7. Physical Inactivity:

Sedentary lifestyles contribute to obesity and insulin resistance, increasing the risk of Type 2 diabetes.

Awareness of these factors is crucial for preventive measures. Lifestyle modifications, such as maintaining a healthy weight, adopting a balanced diet, and regular physical activity, play pivotal roles in diabetes prevention.

GENETIC FACTORS IN DIABETES MELLITUS

Diabetes mellitus, a complex metabolic disorder, has genetic factors playing a pivotal role in its development. While environmental factors like diet and lifestyle contribute significantly, an individual's genetic makeup can predispose them to diabetes. Researchers have identified numerous genetic variants associated with both type 1 and type 2 diabetes.

In type 1 diabetes, an autoimmune condition, specific genetic markers increase susceptibility. Variations in the human leukocyte antigen (HLA) region, particularly HLA-DQ and HLA-DR genes, are strongly linked to type 1 diabetes risk. Additionally, certain non-HLA genes, such as INS and PTPN22, contribute to the genetic component. Type 2 diabetes, more closely tied to lifestyle factors, also exhibits a hereditary component. Family studies and twin studies have shown a higher concordance rate for type 2 diabetes among identical twins compared to non-identical twins. Specific gene variants related to insulin resistance, pancreatic beta-cell function, and glucose metabolism, like those in TCF7L2 and KCNJ11, have been identified as risk factors. Understanding these genetic factors not only aids in identifying individuals at higher risk but also opens avenues for personalized medicine and targeted interventions to mitigate diabetes risk based on an individual's genetic profile.

LIFESTYLE AND ENVIRONMENTAL FACTORS IN DIABETES MELLITUS

Diabetes mellitus, a multifaceted metabolic disorder, is profoundly influenced by lifestyle and environmental factors. In the case of type 2 diabetes, lifestyle choices play a predominant role. Sedentary behavior and inadequate physical activity contribute to obesity, a major risk factor for insulin resistance and diabetes. Unhealthy dietary patterns, high in refined sugars and saturated fats, further exacerbate the risk, influencing weight gain and metabolic dysfunction. Environmental factors, such as urbanization and globalization, have led to shifts in dietary habits and reduced physical activity, contributing to the rising prevalence of diabetes worldwide. Additionally, exposure to environmental toxins and pollutants has been implicated in insulin resistance and diabetes development. Endocrine-disrupting chemicals, found in some plastics and pollutants, may interfere with hormonal regulation, impacting glucose metabolism.

Socioeconomic factors also play a role, as access to healthy foods and opportunities for physical activity can be influenced by economic status. Stress, a common feature of modern lifestyles, can contribute to insulin resistance and exacerbate diabetes risk.

Addressing diabetes requires a holistic approach that considers lifestyle modifications and environmental factors. Public health initiatives promoting healthier diets, increased physical activity, and environmental awareness are crucial components in the global effort to prevent and manage diabetes.

OTHER CONTRIBUTING FACTORS IN DIABETES MELLITUS

Beyond genetic predisposition and lifestyle choices, several other contributing factors impact the development and progression of diabetes mellitus. Age is a significant factor, as the risk of diabetes generally increases with advancing age, particularly in type 2 diabetes. Hormonal influences, such as those related to pregnancy (gestational diabetes) or specific endocrine disorders, can also contribute to diabetes development.

Individuals with certain medical conditions, such as polycystic ovary syndrome (PCOS) or acromegaly, may have an elevated risk of diabetes due to hormonal imbalances. Chronic inflammation, a hallmark of conditions like rheumatoid arthritis, may also play a role in insulin resistance.

Furthermore, medications like corticosteroids and certain antipsychotics can induce insulin resistance, contributing to diabetes onset. Sleep disorders, such as sleep apnea, have been linked to an increased risk of diabetes, possibly due to their impact on metabolic regulation.

Importantly, ethnicity and race are additional factors influencing diabetes risk. Some populations, including African Americans, Hispanics, and Native Americans, exhibit a higher predisposition to diabetes.

Understandings and addressing these diverse contributing factors are essential for comprehensive diabetes prevention and management strategies, highlighting the intricate interplay of biological, environmental, and socio-cultural elements in the development of this pervasive metabolic disorder.

LIVING HEALTHY WITH DIABETES

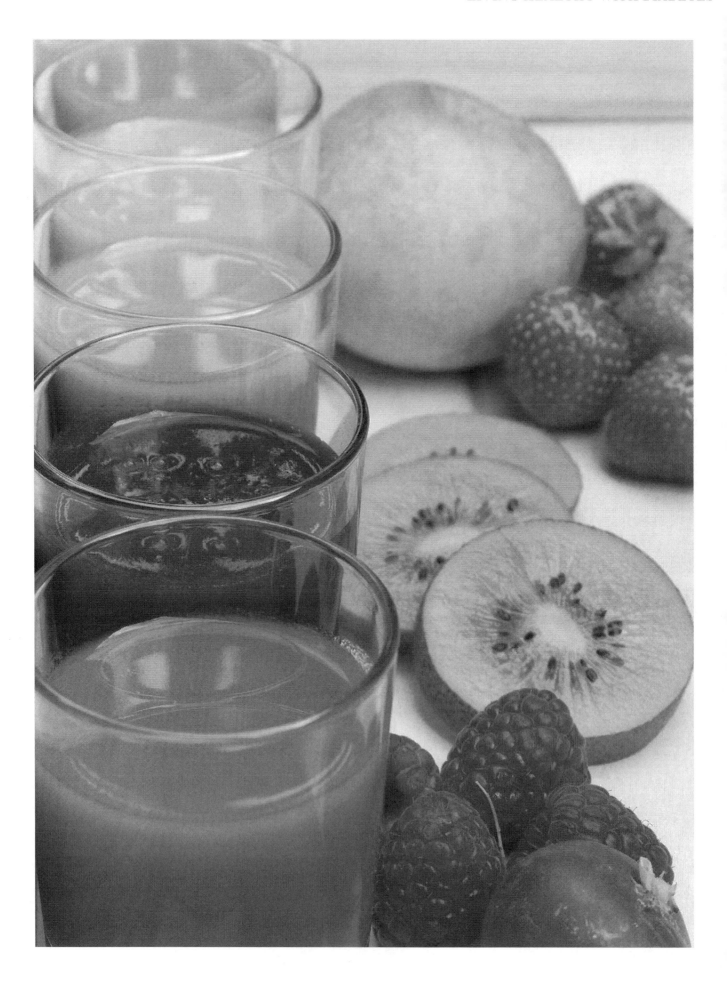

CHAPTER FOUR

RECOGNIZING THE ENEMY: SYMPTOMS AND DIAGNOSIS OF DIABETES MELLITUS

Diabetes, a chronic metabolic disorder, manifests through a range of symptoms that can significantly impact one's health. One prominent sign is increased thirst, known as polydipsia, often accompanied by excessive urination, or polyuria. This occurs as the body tries to eliminate excess glucose through urine. Unexplained weight loss can also be a red flag, despite normal or increased food intake, indicating the body's inability to properly utilize glucose for energy.

Fatigue, a pervasive symptom, stems from cells' inability to receive sufficient glucose, leaving the body drained. Additionally, blurred vision may result from fluctuations in blood sugar levels affecting the eye's lens. Slow wound healing and frequent infections are common due to compromised immune function associated with diabetes.

Individuals might experience tingling or numbness in extremities, a condition known as diabetic neuropathy. Elevated blood sugar levels over time can damage nerves, leading to sensory issues. Furthermore, increased hunger, or polyphagia, may arise as cells crave energy due to ineffective glucose utilization.

It's crucial to recognize these symptoms and seek medical advice promptly. Early diagnosis and management are paramount in controlling diabetes, preventing complications, and promoting overall well-being. Regular monitoring, lifestyle modifications, and, if necessary, medication can help individuals lead healthier lives despite this chronic condition.

THE COMMON SYMPTOMS OF DIABETES MELLITUS

The common symptoms of diabetes mellitus arise from the body's inability to regulate blood glucose effectively. These symptoms may vary in intensity and can manifest differently in Type 1 and Type 2 diabetes. Key indicators include:

1. Excessive Thirst and Hunger:

Increased thirst (polydipsia) and hunger (polyphagia) result from the body's attempt to compensate for elevated blood glucose levels.

2. Frequent Urination:

Excess glucose in the bloodstream prompts the kidneys to work harder to filter and remove it, leading to increased urination (polyuria).

3. Unexplained Weight Loss:

Despite increased appetite, individuals may experience weight loss due to the body utilizing muscle and fat for energy when glucose cannot be adequately absorbed into cells.

4. Fatigue and Weakness:

Inadequate glucose uptake by cells can result in fatigue and weakness, as the body lacks its primary energy source.

5. Blurred Vision:

High blood glucose levels can affect the fluid balance in the eye, leading to blurred vision.

6. Slow Wound Healing:

Impaired circulation and compromised immune function may cause delays in wound healing and increase the risk of infections.

7. Numbness or Tingling:

Prolonged high blood sugar levels can damage nerves, leading to peripheral neuropathy and sensations of numbness or tingling in the extremities.

8. Recurrent Infections:

Increased glucose levels provide an ideal environment for bacterial and fungal growth, making individuals with diabetes more prone to infections.

Recognizing these symptoms is crucial for early diagnosis and intervention. Individuals experiencing these signs should seek medical attention for proper evaluation and management of diabetes mellitus.

THE DIAGNOSTIC TESTS FOR DIABETES MELLITUS

Diagnostic tests for diabetes mellitus involve assessing blood glucose levels to determine the body's ability to regulate sugar. The primary tests include fasting blood sugar (FBS), oral glucose tolerance test (OGTT), and hemoglobin A1c (HbA1c). FBS measures glucose after an overnight fast, with elevated levels suggesting impaired fasting glucose or diabetes. OGTT evaluates the body's response to a glucose load, useful for identifying gestational diabetes or impaired glucose tolerance. HbA1c reflects average blood sugar levels over several months, aiding in long-term diabetes management.

Accurate diagnosis relies on careful interpretation of results, considering individual health factors and potential interferences. Elevated glucose levels alone may not confirm diabetes; repetition and additional tests may be necessary for a conclusive diagnosis.

These diagnostic tools enable healthcare professionals to tailor treatment plans and monitor patients effectively. Early detection through these tests is crucial for timely intervention, preventing complications associated with uncontrolled diabetes. Regular monitoring, lifestyle adjustments, and medication can contribute to effective diabetes management, promoting overall health and well-being.

CHAPTER FIVE

THE COMPLICATIONS OF DIABETES MELLITUS

SHORT TERM COMPLICATIONS

Short-term complications of diabetes mellitus can arise when blood glucose levels become imbalanced, requiring prompt attention to prevent more severe consequences. Hypoglycemia, or low blood sugar, is a common immediate complication. It can result from excessive insulin, insufficient food intake, or increased physical activity. Symptoms include dizziness, confusion, and, if severe, can lead to unconsciousness.

Conversely, hyperglycemia, or high blood sugar, is another short-term complication that may occur when insulin is insufficient to regulate glucose effectively. This can lead to diabetic ketoacidosis (DKA) in type 1 diabetes, causing symptoms like nausea, vomiting, and fruity-smelling breath. In type 2 diabetes, hyperglycemic hyperosmolar state (HHS) may occur, characterized by extreme dehydration and mental status changes.

Additionally, infections can exacerbate blood sugar fluctuations, and individuals with diabetes are more prone to conditions like urinary tract infections and skin infections. These short-term complications highlight the importance of vigilant glucose monitoring, adherence to medication regimens, and timely medical intervention. Education on recognizing and managing these complications is crucial for individuals with diabetes to maintain optimal health and prevent more severe long-term consequences.

LONG TERM COMPLICATIONS

Long-term complications of diabetes mellitus can manifest over years and significantly impact various organ systems. Chronic hyperglycemia can lead to macrovascular complications, contributing to a higher risk of heart disease, stroke, and peripheral vascular disease. It accelerates atherosclerosis, narrowing blood vessels and impairing circulation.

Microvascular complications involve damage to small blood vessels, leading to conditions such as diabetic nephropathy, affecting the kidneys, and diabetic retinopathy, impacting the eyes. Both can progress to severe complications, including kidney failure and blindness, respectively. Neuropathy, affecting nerves throughout the body, is another long-term consequence, causing symptoms ranging from tingling and numbness to pain and impaired organ function.

Foot complications, often related to neuropathy and reduced blood flow, can lead to infections and, in severe cases, amputations. Diabetes also poses a risk for dental issues, skin conditions, and hearing impairment.

Effective management of diabetes, including blood sugar control, lifestyle modifications, and regular medical check-ups, is crucial in preventing or delaying these long-term complications. Patient education, early detection, and comprehensive healthcare support contribute to mitigating the impact of diabetes on overall health and improving the quality of life for individuals living with the condition.

CHAPTER SIX

MANAGEMENT AND TREATMENT FOR DIABETES

The management and treatment of diabetes mellitus involve a multifaceted approach aimed at controlling blood glucose levels, preventing complications, and enhancing overall well-being. Lifestyle modifications play a pivotal role, including a balanced diet, regular physical activity, and maintaining a healthy weight. Monitoring carbohydrate intake and choosing foods with a low glycemic index can help stabilize blood sugar levels.

Medication is often a crucial component of diabetes management. Insulin therapy may be prescribed for type 1 diabetes, and it can be used in conjunction with oral medications for type 2 diabetes. Oral medications such as metformin, sulfonylureas, and others help regulate blood glucose levels through various mechanisms.

Frequent blood glucose monitoring is essential to track fluctuations and make necessary adjustments to the treatment plan. Continuous glucose monitoring (CGM) systems provide real-time data, enhancing precision in managing diabetes.

Patient education is paramount, empowering individuals to make informed decisions about their health. This includes understanding medication regimens, recognizing symptoms of hypo- and hyperglycemia, and adopting a proactive approach to lifestyle choices.

Regular medical check-ups enable healthcare professionals to assess the effectiveness of the treatment plan, monitor for complications, and adjust medications as needed. The collaborative effort between healthcare providers and individuals with diabetes is vital for successful long-term management, promoting a healthy and fulfilling life despite the challenges of the condition.

MEDICATIONS

Medications for diabetes mellitus encompass a diverse array of options designed to regulate blood glucose levels and improve insulin function. In type 1 diabetes, where the body doesn't produce insulin, insulin therapy is essential and may involve rapid-acting, short-acting, intermediate-acting, or long-acting insulin formulations. These are administered via injections or insulin pumps.

For type 2 diabetes, various oral medications and injectables aim to enhance insulin sensitivity, reduce glucose production in the liver, or increase insulin secretion. Metformin, a common first-line oral medication, helps lower blood sugar and improve insulin utilization. Sulfonylureas stimulate insulin release, while thiazolidinediones enhance insulin sensitivity.

Incretin-based therapies, including GLP-1 receptor agonists and DPP-4 inhibitors, regulate blood sugar by affecting gut hormones that influence insulin release. SGLT2 inhibitors promote glucose excretion through urine.

In some cases, healthcare providers may prescribe combination therapies to address multiple aspects of diabetes pathophysiology. Individualized treatment plans consider factors like comorbidities, patient preferences, and potential side effects.

It's crucial for individuals taking diabetes medications to adhere to prescribed regimens, monitor blood glucose levels regularly, and communicate effectively with healthcare providers to optimize treatment. Medication adjustments may be necessary over time to accommodate changing needs and ensure effective diabetes management.

INSULIN THERAPY

Insulin therapy is a cornerstone in the management of diabetes mellitus, particularly for individuals with type 1 diabetes and those with advanced type 2 diabetes where oral medications may not provide adequate control. Insulin, a hormone produced by the pancreas, regulates blood sugar levels by facilitating the uptake of glucose into cells for energy.

For individuals with type 1 diabetes, where the pancreas doesn't produce insulin, and some with type 2 diabetes, exogenous insulin is administered. Various types of insulin exist, classified based on their onset, peak, and duration of action. Rapid-acting insulin is taken just before meals to manage postprandial spikes, while long-acting insulin provides a baseline level throughout the day.

Insulin can be administered through injections using syringes, insulin pens, or insulin pumps. Continuous glucose monitoring (CGM) systems may complement insulin therapy, offering real-time insights to guide dosage adjustments.

Individualized insulin regimens are tailored to factors like lifestyle, eating habits, and activity levels. Intensive insulin therapy, which involves multiple daily injections or continuous subcutaneous insulin infusion, aims for tighter blood glucose control.

Although effective, insulin therapy requires careful monitoring to prevent hypoglycemia (low blood sugar) and optimize glycemic control. Patient education is paramount, empowering individuals to manage insulin dosages, understand injection techniques, and respond to changing insulin needs, promoting a balanced and healthy lifestyle.

LIFESTYLE CHANGES

Lifestyle changes are fundamental in managing diabetes mellitus, playing a pivotal role in controlling blood glucose levels and preventing complications. Dietary modifications are key, emphasizing a well-balanced, low-glycemic index diet that includes whole grains, lean proteins, fruits, and vegetables. Portion control and regular meal timings contribute to stable blood sugar levels.

Regular physical activity is crucial for diabetes management, enhancing insulin sensitivity and promoting weight control. Both aerobic exercises, like walking or cycling, and resistance training are beneficial. Exercise plans should align with individual fitness levels and health conditions.

Maintaining a healthy weight is closely linked to diabetes control. Weight loss, if needed, can significantly improve insulin sensitivity and glycemic control. Additionally, avoiding tobacco and limiting alcohol intake are vital components of a diabetes-friendly lifestyle.

Consistent monitoring of blood glucose levels is essential, providing valuable insights into the effectiveness of lifestyle changes and allowing for timely adjustments. Stress management techniques, such as meditation or yoga, can also contribute to overall well-being.

Regular medical check-ups ensure that healthcare providers can assess the impact of lifestyle changes, make necessary adjustments to treatment plans, and address any emerging issues. Patient education is paramount, empowering individuals to make informed choices about their lifestyle, promoting long-term health and reducing the risk of diabetes-related complications.

LIVING HEALTHY WITH DIABETES

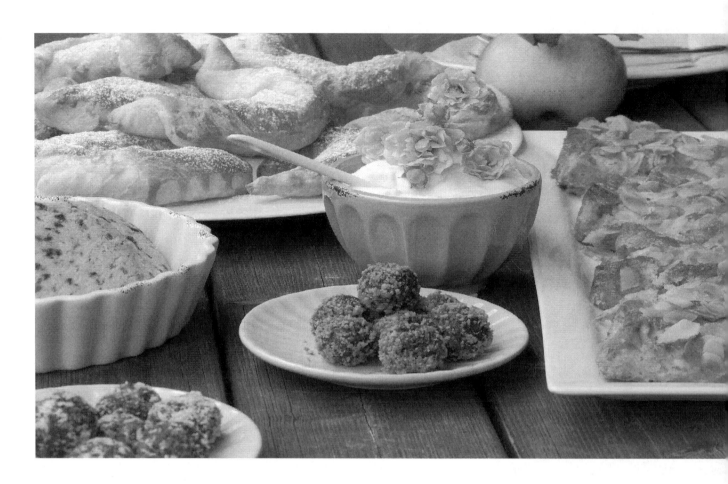

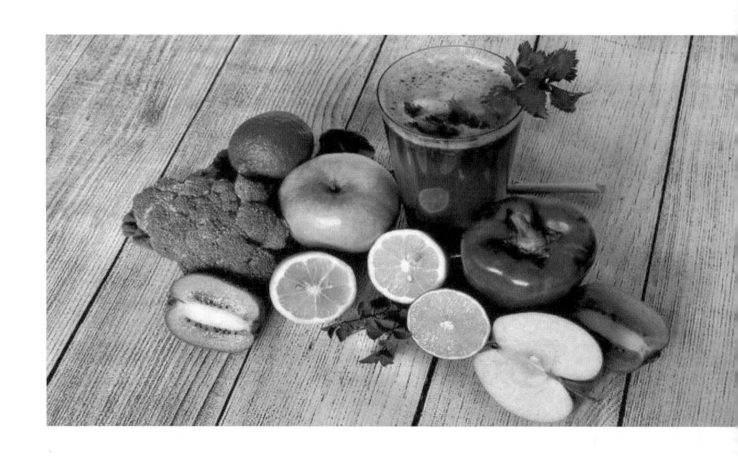

CHAPTER SEVEN

DIET AND NUTRITION FOR DIABETES MELLITUS

Diet and nutrition play a central role in managing diabetes mellitus, influencing blood glucose levels and overall health. A balanced diet that considers the glycemic index of foods is crucial. Choosing complex carbohydrates, such as whole grains, legumes, and vegetables, helps regulate blood sugar levels by providing a steady release of glucose.

Portion control is essential to prevent overeating and large spikes in blood sugar. Incorporating lean proteins, like poultry, fish, and tofu, supports satiety and helps maintain muscle mass. Healthy fats from sources like avocados, nuts, and olive oil are beneficial, but portion sizes should be monitored.

Fruits can be included in the diet, but moderation is key due to their natural sugars. Monitoring carbohydrate intake and spacing meals evenly throughout the day contribute to glycemic control.

Individualized meal planning is crucial, considering factors like age, activity level, and any concurrent health conditions. Regular monitoring of blood glucose levels aids in understanding how different foods impact individual responses.

Working with a registered dietitian or healthcare professional can provide personalized guidance. Additionally, staying hydrated and limiting the intake of sugary beverages is important.

Overall, a well-rounded, nutritious diet not only helps manage blood glucose levels but also supports weight management, cardiovascular health, and overall well-being for individuals with diabetes.

IMPORTANCE OF HEALTHY EATING IN DIABETES MELLITUS

Maintaining a healthy diet is paramount for individuals with diabetes mellitus as it significantly influences blood sugar levels and overall well-being. Proper nutrition empowers individuals to manage their condition effectively, minimizing the risk of complications. Controlling carbohydrate intake is a cornerstone, as carbohydrates directly impact blood glucose levels. Opting for complex carbohydrates with a low glycemic index, such as whole grains and legumes, helps regulate blood sugar.

Furthermore, the inclusion of fiber in the diet aids in digestion and slows the absorption of sugar, promoting more stable blood glucose levels. Healthy fats, like those found in avocados and nuts, can contribute to heart health, crucial for diabetics who often face an increased risk of cardiovascular issues. Monitoring portion sizes is essential, preventing overconsumption of calories that can lead to weight gain—another factor influencing diabetes management.

Beyond glucose control, a balanced diet supports overall health, bolstering the immune system and reducing the risk of complications related to diabetes, such as nerve damage and kidney disease. Making informed food choices, limiting processed sugars, and maintaining a consistent eating schedule are integral components of a holistic approach to diabetes care. In essence, embracing healthy eating habits empowers individuals with diabetes to lead fuller, healthier lives while effectively managing their condition.

MEAL PLANNING FOR DIABETICS

Effective meal planning is a cornerstone of managing diabetes, providing individuals with the tools to regulate blood sugar levels and maintain overall health. The key lies in creating well-balanced meals that control carbohydrates, incorporate lean proteins, and include healthy fats. Distributing carbohydrate intake throughout the day helps prevent spikes in blood sugar, promoting stability.

In meal planning for diabetics, selecting foods with a low glycemic index is crucial. This includes whole grains, vegetables, and legumes, as they have a slower impact on blood sugar levels. Portion control is equally vital to avoid overloading the body with excessive calories and carbohydrates. Consistency in meal timing is also beneficial, helping to regulate insulin levels and promote steady glucose levels.

The inclusion of fiber-rich foods aids digestion and contributes to satiety, preventing overeating. Additionally, incorporating lean proteins, such as poultry, fish, and tofu, supports muscle health and helps manage weight.

Individualized meal plans, developed in consultation with healthcare professionals or dietitians, consider factors like age, activity level, and personal preferences. Regular monitoring of blood sugar levels enables adjustments to the meal plan as needed, ensuring optimal diabetes management. Ultimately, a well-thought-out and personalized meal plan empowers individuals with diabetes to make informed and healthy food choices, promoting better overall well-being.

GLYCEMIC INDEX AND GLYCEMIC LOAD

The glycemic index (GI) and glycemic load (GL) are important concepts in understanding how different foods affect blood sugar levels. The glycemic index measures how quickly a carbohydrate-containing food raises blood glucose levels compared to a reference food (usually glucose or white bread). Foods with a high GI cause a rapid spike in blood sugar, while those with a low GI result in a slower, more gradual increase.

On the other hand, glycemic load takes into account both the quality and quantity of carbohydrates in a specific serving of food. It provides a more comprehensive picture by considering the actual amount of carbohydrates consumed. A food with a high glycemic index may have a lower glycemic load if the total carbohydrates per serving are low.

Choosing foods with a low GI and managing glycemic load is particularly beneficial for individuals with diabetes. A diet emphasizing low-GI foods can help control blood sugar levels and reduce the risk of complications. However, it's important to note that these concepts are just one aspect of a healthy diet, and overall nutritional balance, portion control, and individualized meal planning are crucial factors in managing diabetes effectively.

CHAPTER EIGHT

THE PHYSICAL ACTIVITIES FOR DIABETICS FOR OPTIMAL RECOVERY

Physical activity is a cornerstone in the management of diabetes, offering a range of benefits that contribute to improved overall health. Regular exercise helps control blood sugar levels by enhancing insulin sensitivity, allowing cells to better utilize glucose. It also aids in weight management, a crucial aspect for individuals with diabetes as excess weight can exacerbate the condition.

Engaging in both aerobic exercises, such as brisk walking or cycling, and resistance training, like weightlifting, provides a comprehensive approach. Aerobic activities improve cardiovascular health, while resistance training enhances muscle strength and metabolism, contributing to better glucose control.

Consistency is key when incorporating physical activity into a diabetic lifestyle. Regular exercise can help reduce the risk of complications associated with diabetes, including heart disease and nerve damage. Additionally, it promotes stress reduction and mental well-being.

Before starting any exercise regimen, individuals with diabetes should consult their healthcare professionals to ensure a safe and suitable plan. Monitoring blood sugar levels before and after exercise helps tailor activities to individual needs. By making physical activity a consistent part of their routine, individuals with diabetes can significantly enhance their overall health and better manage their condition.

EXERCISE RECOMMENDATIONS FOR DIABETICS

Exercise is a crucial component of diabetes management, offering a multitude of benefits for individuals with the condition. The American Diabetes Association recommends at least 150 minutes of moderate-intensity aerobic exercise per week, spread across at least three days, for adults with diabetes. This can include activities like brisk walking, cycling, or swimming. Alternatively, engaging in 75 minutes of vigorous-intensity aerobic exercise is another effective option.

In addition to aerobic exercises, incorporating strength training exercises at least two days per week is advised. This could involve weightlifting, resistance band exercises, or bodyweight exercises. Strength training helps build muscle mass, improves insulin sensitivity, and contributes to better overall metabolic health.

Flexibility and balance exercises are also beneficial, reducing the risk of falls, particularly important for older individuals with diabetes.

Individuals with diabetes should tailor their exercise routine to their preferences and health status, with a focus on consistency. Regular monitoring of blood sugar levels before and after exercise helps in adjusting medications and managing potential fluctuations.

Before initiating a new exercise program, consulting with healthcare professionals is essential, especially for those with existing health concerns. Customizing exercise plans based on individual needs ensures that physical activity becomes a safe and enjoyable part of diabetes management.

BENEFIT OF REGULAR PHYSICAL ACTIVITY

Physical activity is particularly advantageous for individuals with diabetes, offering a spectrum of benefits that contribute to improved health and better management of the condition. One of the primary advantages is enhanced blood sugar control. Regular exercise improves insulin sensitivity, allowing cells to more efficiently utilize glucose, thus helping to regulate blood sugar levels.

Engaging in physical activity is pivotal for weight management, a critical aspect for individuals with diabetes, as excess weight can exacerbate the condition. Exercise aids in maintaining a healthy body weight, reducing the risk of complications associated with diabetes.

Moreover, regular physical activity has a positive impact on cardiovascular health, lowering the risk of heart disease—a prevalent concern for those with diabetes. It improves circulation, lowers blood pressure, and contributes to healthier cholesterol levels.

Exercise also plays a role in stress reduction, promoting mental well-being. It releases endorphins, reducing symptoms of anxiety and depression, which can be more prevalent in individuals managing chronic conditions like diabetes.

Consistency is key, and incorporating a variety of exercises, including aerobic activities and strength training, offers a comprehensive approach. Before starting any exercise regimen, individuals with diabetes should consult healthcare professionals to tailor a plan that suits their specific needs and health status. Ultimately, the benefits of regular physical activity for diabetics extend beyond glucose control, encompassing overall health and well-being.

CHAPTER NINE

MONITORING BLOOD SUGAR LEVELS

Monitoring blood sugar levels is a crucial aspect of diabetes management, providing valuable information to help individuals make informed decisions about their treatment plan and lifestyle. Here are key points about monitoring blood sugar levels in diabetics:

1. Frequency:

The frequency of monitoring can vary depending on the individual's type of diabetes, treatment plan, and overall health. Some may need to check several times a day, while others may check less frequently.

2.Methods:

Blood sugar levels are typically measured using a blood glucose meter. A small drop of blood, usually obtained by pricking the fingertip, is placed on a test strip, and the meter provides a reading.

3 Timing:

Monitoring at different times of the day offers a comprehensive view. This includes fasting levels in the morning, before and after meals, and sometimes before bedtime.

4 Target Ranges:

Healthcare professionals often set target blood sugar ranges for individuals. These targets may vary based on factors like age, duration of diabetes, and overall health.

5 Adjustments:

Monitoring helps individuals and healthcare providers make adjustments to medication, diet, and physical activity to maintain optimal blood sugar control.

6 Continuous Glucose Monitoring (CGM):

Some individuals use CGM systems, which provide real-time information about glucose levels throughout the day. CGM can offer a more detailed and continuous picture of blood sugar trends.

Regular monitoring empowers individuals with diabetes to proactively manage their condition, minimizing the risk of complications and promoting overall well-being. It's essential for individuals to work closely with their healthcare team to determine the most effective monitoring routine for their specific needs.

HOME MONITORING

Home monitoring of blood sugar levels is a fundamental and empowering aspect of diabetes management, enabling individuals to take an active role in their health. Utilizing a blood glucose meter at home provides real-time insights into how the body processes glucose, helping individuals make timely adjustments to their lifestyle and treatment plans.

The process involves a small, relatively painless prick to the fingertip to obtain a drop of blood. This blood is then applied to a test strip inserted into a glucose meter. Within seconds, the meter provides a numerical reading of the blood sugar level. Home monitoring allows individuals to check their blood sugar at various times, such as fasting in the morning, before and after meals, and before bedtime.

Regular monitoring empowers individuals to understand how their activities, meals, and medications impact blood sugar levels. It facilitates proactive management, enabling prompt adjustments to medication dosages, dietary choices, and exercise routines. Additionally, it serves as a valuable tool for healthcare professionals, offering them comprehensive data to make informed decisions about the individual's treatment plan during regular check-ups.

Continuous advancements, including the use of mobile apps and connectivity features, further enhance the convenience and effectiveness of home blood sugar monitoring, fostering a more personalized and responsive approach to diabetes care.

IMPORTANCE OF REGULAR CHECKS

Regular blood sugar level checks are of paramount importance in managing diabetes effectively and preventing complications associated with the condition. Monitoring blood sugar levels provides critical insights into how the body processes glucose, allowing individuals and healthcare professionals to make informed decisions about treatment and lifestyle adjustments.

By checking blood sugar levels regularly, individuals can identify patterns and trends, understanding how factors such as meals, physical activity, and medication impact their glucose levels. This knowledge enables them to make timely adjustments, optimizing blood sugar control and reducing the risk of hyperglycemia (high blood sugar) or hypoglycemia (low blood sugar).

Consistent monitoring is crucial for adjusting medication dosages. For those on insulin or oral medications, understanding how their current regimen aligns with their blood sugar patterns helps prevent overmedication or inadequate control. This personalized approach enhances the effectiveness of the treatment plan, promoting better overall health.

Regular checks also serve as an early warning system, allowing for prompt intervention if blood sugar levels deviate from target ranges.

This proactive management can help prevent long-term complications such as cardiovascular disease, kidney problems, and nerve damage.

In essence, the importance of regular blood sugar level checks lies in their role as a proactive tool for personalized diabetes management, facilitating informed decision-making and contributing to the overall well-being of individuals living with diabetes.

CHAPTER TEN

PSYCHOSOCIAL ASPECTS OF DIABETES

The psychosocial aspects of diabetes mellitus encompass a wide array of social and psychological factors that influence an individual's experience of living with the condition.

1. Social Support:

The support system plays a crucial role in diabetes management. Positive interactions with family, friends, and healthcare professionals can contribute significantly to emotional well-being and adherence to treatment plans. Conversely, lack of understanding or support may lead to feelings of isolation and frustration.

2. Stigma and Discrimination:

Stigma surrounding diabetes can impact individuals psychologically. Misconceptions about the causes of diabetes may contribute to feelings of blame or shame. Discrimination in various settings, including workplaces or social gatherings, can exacerbate these negative emotions.

3. Quality of Life:

Diabetes can affect various aspects of daily life, influencing factors such as work, relationships, and recreational activities. Balancing these aspects while managing the demands of diabetes requires ongoing adaptation and resilience.

4. Cultural and Economic Factors:

Cultural beliefs and socioeconomic status can influence how individuals perceive and manage diabetes. Access to healthcare resources, cultural norms, and economic factors may impact treatment adherence and health outcomes.

Addressing the psychosocial aspects of diabetes requires a comprehensive approach that includes education, counseling, and community support. Recognizing and mitigating the psychosocial challenges individuals face is essential for fostering a holistic and patient-centered approach to diabetes care.

EMOTIONAL ASPECTS OF DIABETES

The emotional impact of diabetes mellitus can be profound, influencing various aspects of an individual's well-being. Diagnosis often brings a range of emotions, including shock, fear, and uncertainty about the future. The chronic nature of the condition can lead to persistent emotional challenges.

1. Anxiety and Stress:

Managing diabetes involves daily monitoring, medication, and lifestyle adjustments. The constant need for vigilance can contribute to heightened anxiety and stress, as individuals navigate the complexities of blood sugar control.

2. Fear of Complications:

Concerns about potential complications, such as cardiovascular issues, neuropathy, and kidney disease, can create a pervasive sense of fear and worry. Regular medical check-ups and communication with healthcare professionals are crucial in addressing and alleviating these concerns.

3. Impact on Relationships:

Diabetes can affect relationships, as partners and family members may also experience emotional strain. Open communication and mutual understanding are vital for navigating the emotional aspects of living with diabetes as a family.

4. Guilt and Shame:

Individuals may experience feelings of guilt or shame, particularly if they perceive themselves as responsible for their diabetes diagnosis.

Educating individuals about the multifactorial nature of diabetes and promoting self-compassion is crucial in addressing these emotions.

5.Coping Strategies:

Developing healthy coping strategies, such as seeking support from healthcare professionals, joining support groups, and incorporating stress-reducing activities into daily life, is essential. Emotional well-being is an integral component of diabetes care, and addressing the emotional impact ensures a holistic approach to managing this chronic condition.

COPING STRATEGIES FOR DIABETES

Coping with diabetes mellitus involves adopting effective strategies to navigate the physical and emotional challenges associated with the condition.

1.Education and Awareness:

Understanding diabetes and its management is a powerful coping strategy. Education empowers individuals to make informed decisions about lifestyle choices, medication adherence, and overall self-care.

2.Social Support:

Building a strong support network is crucial. Family, friends, and support groups provide emotional encouragement and practical assistance. Sharing experiences with others who have diabetes can alleviate feelings of isolation and offer valuable insights.

3.Healthy Lifestyle Habits:

Adopting and maintaining a healthy lifestyle significantly contributes to diabetes management. This includes a balanced diet, regular physical activity, sufficient sleep, and stress-reducing activities. These habits not only help control blood sugar levels but also contribute to overall well-being.

4.Mindfulness and Stress Management:

Practices such as mindfulness meditation, deep breathing exercises, and yoga can help manage stress, which is closely linked to diabetes management. Stress reduction techniques contribute to better emotional health and improved blood sugar control.

5. Regular Monitoring and Communication:

Consistent blood sugar monitoring allows for proactive management. Regular communication with healthcare professionals ensures that treatment plans are optimized based on individual needs and changing circumstances.

6. Adaptability and Resilience:

Diabetes management requires adaptability. Individuals who develop resilience in the face of challenges are better equipped to navigate the ups and downs associated with living with a chronic condition.

Coping strategies are highly individualized, and finding what works best often involves a combination of these approaches. Regularly reassessing and adjusting coping strategies based on evolving needs ensures ongoing effective diabetes management.

CHAPTER ELEVEN

PREVENTION AND RISK REDUCTION OF DIABETES

Preventive measures for diabetes mellitus revolve around lifestyle modifications that target key risk factors associated with the development of the condition.

1. Healthy Eating Habits:

Adopting a balanced and nutrient-rich diet is fundamental. Emphasizing whole foods, limiting refined sugars and processed foods, and controlling portion sizes contribute to weight management and glucose control.

2. Regular Physical Activity:

Incorporating regular exercise into daily routines is a cornerstone of diabetes prevention. Both aerobic activities, like brisk walking or cycling, and strength training enhance insulin sensitivity and promote overall health.

3. Weight Management:

Maintaining a healthy weight significantly reduces the risk of diabetes. Even modest weight loss in overweight individuals can have a substantial impact on preventing the onset of the disease.

4. Avoiding Sedentary Lifestyle:

Limiting sedentary behavior, such as prolonged sitting, is crucial. Breaking up long periods of inactivity with short bouts of movement can improve insulin sensitivity.

5. Monitoring Blood Sugar Levels:

Regular monitoring of blood sugar levels, especially for individuals with risk factors, allows for early detection and intervention. This is particularly important for those with prediabetes, as lifestyle changes can often reverse this condition.

6. Regular Health Check-ups:

Periodic health check-ups, including blood pressure and cholesterol monitoring, aid in identifying and managing risk factors associated with diabetes.

Preventive measures should be individualized based on risk factors, and early intervention through lifestyle changes remains a powerful strategy in averting the onset of diabetes mellitus. Public health initiatives focusing on education and promoting healthy lifestyles further contribute to broader preventive efforts.

CHAPTER TWELVE

LIVING WITH DIABETES: OVERCOMING DAILY CHALLENGES

Living with diabetes mellitus is a lifelong journey that involves daily self-care, making informed choices, and adapting to the challenges associated with managing the condition.

1. Blood Sugar Management:

Regular monitoring of blood sugar levels is essential for individuals with diabetes. This involves checking levels before and after meals, adjusting medications as needed, and being vigilant about signs of hyperglycemia or hypoglycemia.

2. Medication Adherence:

Depending on the type of diabetes, individuals may need to take medications such as insulin or oral medications. Adhering to prescribed medication regimens is critical for maintaining optimal blood sugar control.

3. Lifestyle Adjustments:

Adopting a healthy lifestyle is foundational. This includes maintaining a balanced diet, engaging in regular physical activity, and managing stress. Lifestyle adjustments contribute not only to blood sugar control but also to overall well-being.

4. Regular Medical Check-ups:

Routine visits to healthcare professionals are vital for monitoring overall health, detecting any complications early, and adjusting treatment plans as needed. Eye examinations, kidney function tests, and cardiovascular assessments are often part of these check-ups.

5. Emotional Well-being:

Managing the emotional impact of diabetes is crucial. Support from family, friends, and healthcare professionals, as well as engaging in stress-reducing activities, contributes to emotional well-being.

6. Continuous Learning:

Staying informed about diabetes, treatment advancements, and self-care practices is an ongoing process. Education empowers individuals to take an active role in their health and make informed decisions.

Living with diabetes requires resilience, adaptability, and a holistic approach to health. With proper management and support, individuals can lead fulfilling lives while effectively managing the challenges associated with diabetes mellitus.

EVERYDAY CHALLENGES

The everyday challenges of living with diabetes mellitus are multifaceted, requiring constant attention and adaptation to maintain optimal health.

1.Dietary Discipline:

Balancing meals, counting carbohydrates, and making mindful food choices pose daily challenges. Individuals with diabetes must navigate social situations, dining out, and unexpected dietary temptations while adhering to nutritional guidelines.

2.Blood Sugar Monitoring:

Regularly checking blood sugar levels involves consistent finger pricking, which can be physically and emotionally taxing. The need for continuous monitoring adds a layer of vigilance to daily activities.

3.Medication Management:

Adhering to medication regimens, whether through insulin injections or oral medications, demands a strict schedule. Managing doses, refilling prescriptions, and ensuring medications are stored appropriately are routine tasks.

4.Physical Activity:

Incorporating regular exercise into daily life requires planning and commitment. Balancing physical activity with potential fluctuations in blood sugar levels adds complexity to maintaining an active lifestyle.

5.Emotional Impact:

The emotional toll of living with a chronic condition is significant. Coping with the fear of complications, potential stigma, and the constant awareness of the condition can contribute to stress, anxiety, and emotional fatigue.

6.Social and Work Situations:

Navigating social events and workplace environments can be challenging. Explaining dietary restrictions, managing medication schedules discreetly, and coping with potential misconceptions about diabetes demand resilience in various social settings.

The cumulative impact of these daily challenges underscores the need for ongoing support, education, and mental health resources to help individuals with diabetes navigate the intricacies of daily life while effectively managing their conditio.

SUPPORT SYSTEMS FOR THOSE LIVING WITH DIABETES

Support systems play a crucial role in helping individuals effectively navigate the challenges of living with diabetes mellitus.

1.Family and Friends:

 A strong support network at home can provide emotional encouragement, understanding, and practical assistance. Family and friends who actively engage in learning about diabetes contribute to creating a supportive environment.

2.Healthcare Professionals:

 Diabetes management is a collaborative effort with healthcare professionals. Regular check-ups, consultations, and access to diabetes educators empower individuals with the knowledge and tools to manage their condition effectively.

3.Support Groups:

Joining diabetes support groups allows individuals to connect with others facing similar challenges. These groups provide a platform for sharing experiences, practical tips, and emotional support, reducing feelings of isolation.

4. Online Communities:

Virtual communities and forums provide a space for individuals to seek advice, share information, and find encouragement from people around the world dealing with diabetes. Online platforms can offer a sense of community and accessibility.

5. Workplace Support:

Employers who promote a supportive workplace environment contribute to the well-being of employees with diabetes. Accommodations for medical appointments, understanding regarding breaks for blood sugar management, and fostering a culture of wellness are essential.

6. Mental Health Professionals:

Managing the emotional impact of diabetes is crucial. Psychologists, counselors, or mental health professionals can provide coping strategies, stress management techniques, and a safe space to discuss the psychological aspects of living with diabetes.

Building and maintaining a robust support system is essential for individuals with diabetes, fostering resilience and enhancing overall well-being as they navigate the complexities of their daily lives.

A MESSAGE OF HOPE DESPITE A JOURNEY WITH DIABETES

Amidst the difficulties presented by Diabetes, a message of hope radiates through. Hope is a strong power that can motivate people and their friends and family to strive on, adjust, and track down satisfaction throughout everyday life. Here is a message of Hope for those on the journey with Diabetes:

Diabetes might bring vulnerability and change, yet it doesn't define what your identity is. Your solidarity, versatility, and the affection and backing of your family and community are sources of boundless Hope.

You are not alone on this journey; a great many people all over the planet are exploring it with you.

Hope dwells in the continuous research and advancements in understanding Diabetes better. Consistently, researchers and medical services experts work indefatigably to further develop therapies, reveal new treatments, and at last find a cure. Your association in research and clinical preliminaries adds to these endeavors.

Each second you embrace existence with Diabetes is a demonstration of your fortitude and determination. It's a reminder that in spite of the difficulties, there is delight to be found, purpose to be fulfilled, and a life well-lived.

Thus, let hope be your aide. With hope, there is strength. With hope, there is progress. With hope, there is the commitment of a more promising time to come. Diabetes might be a piece of your journeys, however it doesn't need to be the sum of it. Embrace existence with hope, for a reference point lights your way towards a seriously satisfying and upbeat tomorrow.

Made in United States
Troutdale, OR
08/31/2024